KRATOM BOOK

Bali Kratom, Thai Kratom, and Maeng da Kratom Information; Kratom for Opioid Addiction Withdrawal and Pain Relief and Anxiety Treatment

Catherine Smith

COPYRIGHT

TABLE OF CONTENT

CHAPTER ONE- INTRODUCTION, SCIENTIFIC CLASSIFICATION AND DESCRIPTION OF KRATOM

INTRODUCTION

Kratom, also known to be ketum is an evergreen tree that originated from Southeast Asia (Indonesia, Malaysia, Borneo, Myanmar, Thailand). Mitragyna speciosa is the botanical name. Coffee tea (Rubiaceae) and kratom are from the same plant family. Its leaves have long been used as herbal drugs by the Southeast Asians. In folk medicines, it serves as sedatives at high doses, stimulants at low doses, painkiller, recreational drugs, medication for opiate addiction and diarrhea. It is also reported that kratom can be used in the treatment of restless legs syndrome (RLS), arthritis, and fibromyalgia.

SCIENTIFIC CLASSIFICATION OF KRATOM

Kingdom: Plantae

Clade: Angiosperms

Clade: Eudicots

Clade: Asterids

Order: Gentianales

Family: Rubiaceae

Genus: Mitragyna

Species: M. speciosa

Binomial name—Mitragyna speciosa

SYNONYMS

Nauclea korthalsii Steud. nom. inval.

Nauclea luzoniensis Blanco

Nauclea speciosa (Korth.) Miq.

Stephegyne speciosa Korth.

DESCRIPTION

Mitragyna speciosa is a tropical evergreen tree which grows to about 25 m (82 ft.) tall with the trunk growing up to a 0.9 m (3 ft.) diameter. The trunk is usually straight, with smooth grey outer bark. The leaves look dark green and glossy, growing to over 7–12 cm (2.8–4.7 in) wide and 14–20 cm (5.5–7.9 in) long when fully open. The leaves have ovate-acuminate shape, and with opposite growth pattern, having 12–17 pairs of veins. At the ends of the branches, the flowers are in clusters of three. The corolla-tube has a length of 2.5–3 millimeters (0.098–0.118 in), while the length of the calyx-tube is 2 mm (0.079 in) with five lobes.

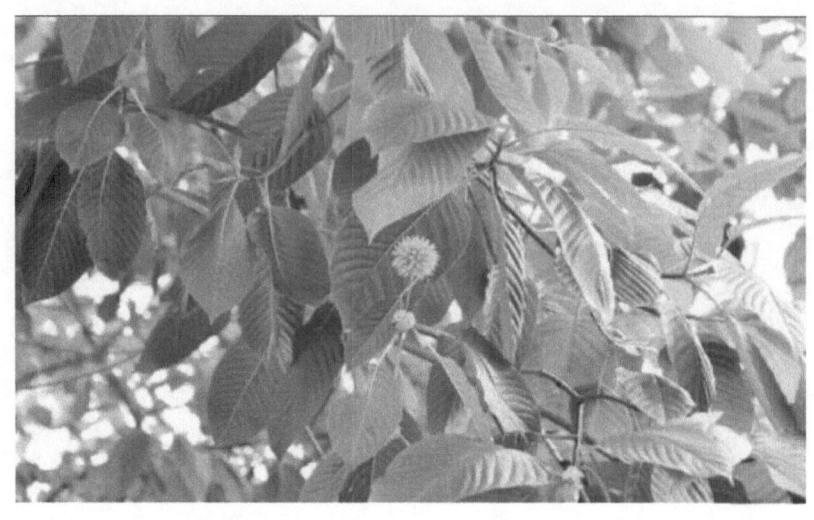

Mitragynine has a lesser analgesic impact compared to morphine. However, it doesn't exactly cause much dependence which makes it a better option for relieving minor to moderate aches and pains. This is one of the reasons why most people get Kratom. Typically, there is a high amount of mitragynine in the plant, which makes it practical to extract. The strongest analgesic effects have been found in 7-hydrohydroxymitrangynine. However, it´s not found in ample quantity in Kratom. It´s not exactly practical to extract this type of alkaloid since its quite rare, however, if the ordinary mitragynine could somehow be converted into 7- hydrohydroxymitrangynine, modern medication could progress manifolds on its basis. People who get Kratom would be able to enjoy a lot of advantages then.

CHAPTER TWO- CHEMISTRY AND PHARMACOLOGY OF KRATOM

CHEMISTRY

There are over 40 compounds found in M. speciosa which include over 25 alkaloids like mitragynine pseudoindoxyl, ajmalicine, Rhynchophylline, and mitraphylline, but the primary psychoactive compounds found are 7-hydroxymitragynine (7-HMG) and mitragynine. Other active compounds present in M. speciosa include Pausinystalia johimbe alkaloids like corynantheidine and raubasine (best known from Rauvolfia serpentina).Mitragynine is composed of about 60% of alkaloid, while 7-hydroxymitragynine alkaloid is about 2%. The structure of Mitragynine is similar to voacangine and yohimbine.

Pharmacology of Kratom

About 20 active elements found in kratom has been shown to be responsible for the pharmacological effects that lead to its benefits to the body. The most characterized active pharmacology agents in kratom are the mitragynine analogs. These agents have an indole ring and are structurally similar to yohimbine. These agents produce a broad variety of pharmacologic effects in vivo and in vitro. The importance of these compounds can be seen in its function as analgesia and an opioid suppressant.

Kratom Analgesic and Opioid-Like Effects

Kratom has been used over the years in Southeast Asia for the treatment of pain and during opium withdrawal, so also is the same in the West.

Evidence proves that kratom, molecules from kratom and kratom extracts can provide different relief forms of pain in animal models. Most of the peripheral and central nervous system effects of these substances derived from kratom are inhibition by opioid antagonists. The opioid-like activity of kratom is connected to the presence of the mitragynine and 7-Hydroxymitragynine and indole alkaloids. Both compounds possess antinociceptive and analgesic effects in animals, but 7-Hydroxymitragynime has more potency than mitragynine. These chemicals also exert opioid-like effects on organs like the male internal genitalia and intestines. When animals were given kratom for five days, the two compounds resulted in a physical dependency state having withdrawal symptoms like the opioids. Also, ligand binding studies, as well as studies that use opioid antagonists, show that the effects are assisted by the actions of δ- and μ-type opioid receptors.

Kratom also possesses an anti-inflammatory effect along with other central nervous system effects. Mitragynine also can inhibit lipopolysaccharide stimulated prostaglandin E2 production and cyclooxygenase-2 expression. It also has antinociceptive effects which may include the stimulation of the descending serotonergic and noradrenergic pathways in the spinal cord. Furthermore, studies have shown that mitragynine can stimulate postsynaptic α2-adrenergic receptor and also, this same compound can lead to blockage of 5-hydroxytryptamine2A receptors. The level of 7-hydroxymitragynine contained in kratom is lower than mitragynine, but it is suggested that7-hydroxymitragynine has more potency and a more significant blood-brain-barrier penetration and oral bioavailability than mitragynine enabling it to be the highest mediator of the analgesic effects kratom has in the body.

Some other compounds like Speciocilliatine, Paynatheine, and Speciogynine are also available in kratom and have some effects as well in the body. These compounds modulate the function and behavioral response of the intestinal smooth muscle in animals.

CHAPTER THREE: BALI KRATOM

Bali Kratom is the powder of dried leaves of Mitrangyna Speciosa. It is a tree found mostly in regions of Southeast Asia. The tree belongs to a similar botanical group to which coffee tree belongs. Kratom is a tree with lots of medicinal properties. Also, the herbal drugs made from this tree are also used in recreational property treatment in humans as well. Also, Bali Kratom leaves are now sold in the market due to their many medicinal advantages and use for the human body.

BALI KRATOM EFFECT AND PRODUCT INFORMATION

Bali Kratom grows in Borneo forests. Bali Kratom is one of the greatest medicines, which can be used for relaxing and energizing the body. Thus if you are feeling your body is running low on energy or if you are feeling tired from several days despite getting all rest, then Bali Kratom can be of great help to you. Bali Kratom is one of the most effective drugs if you are searching for drugs to relax your body down. Moreover, being a superior relaxing drug, it can also be utilized as mood enhancer as well.

Bali Kratom as it is known for its lots of medicinal properties. It is a drug good for easing down pain. Thus if you are suffering from injury or internal body pain, Bali Kratom can be great pain relievers. Moreover, the herb is also helpful in dealing with stress and depression problems. Many doctors have claimed success dealing with stress-related and depression related problems with Bali Kratom.

Moreover, if you are a person who gets hype very quickly or loses temper quickly, then also Bali Kratom is of great help to you. It keeps you calm and cool from the mind. Once consumed you can feel the calmness running in your body, and you might like to listen to some music desperately. Thus keeping Bali Kratom advantages in mind, one can say it as a drug with more analgesic property.

Despite being a drug with so many positives for the human body, Bali Kratom is not an addictive drug. However, one must consider several things before consuming this drug. Things such as Bali Kratom effects are temporary and may disappear after several days. For example, if you used this drug once to get rid of pain or to feel energized then the effects may last for several days and in some cases several hours. Moreover, Bali Kratom is good for utilization over synthetic drugs that come with a lever damage danger.

Despite being a drug which hardly is addictive, if one still gets addicted towards it, then it is not the drug with as a harmful effect as heroin or codeine. Kratom must be considered solely. If Kratom is consumed with other drugs, then it can be a lot more dangerous. Also, Kratom is dangerous if consumed with things such as alcohol or so on.

It is always necessary to take Bali Kratom if suggested by a specialist doctor. Moreover, one must consume a specific amount of dosage of this drug. As the drug helps in relaxing and energizing the body, chances for anyone to fall asleep are high. Thus using Kratom when you are about to drive is not at all recommended.

CHAPTER FOUR: KRATOM PILLS

Kratom pills are made of kratom herbs, a popular medicinal plant that is common in the Asian continent. The tree leaves have been used for centuries to cure various maladies more so in the oriental countries such as Thailand and Malaysia where Kratom trees are mostly found. The extract is currently availed in descent palatable forms such in capsule or in powder form. Presently, this medicinal plant is available in conventional medical stores due to its efficacy after being used for a while yielding positive results. Some clinical studies and trials have confirmed the positive pharmacological effects of kratom pills.

The kratom extracts contain an epicatechin a powerful oxidant that has been identified as effective in eradicating free radicals in the blood circulation system. The oxidant helps to inhibit activities of carcinogenic cells hence, reduce cancer chances in frequents users of the pill. The alkaloid contained in this medicinal product is also effective in boosting the body immune system. For those working long hours or overnight, the pill is a good stimulant that will keep awake the whole night without worrying about addictions.

Some of the clinicians have found the kratom pills useful in the management of adverse pain as it exhibits properties similar to caffeine. The pills are comparatively to nonaddictive compared to caffeine derivatives. Also, Kratom pills are effective in the management of opiate addiction. The pill helps in the reduction of craving of addictive substances helping the addicts to recover from addiction. The pill has found its way in drug rehab as it provides a non-addictive alternative for those under rehabilitation. Additionally, the pill is effective in the treatment of sleep disturbances. Hence, it's an exceptional sedative. Other conditions that the Kraton pill is used to manage are:

1) Anxiety

2) Depression

3) Fatigue

4) Body aches

5) Chronic insomnia

6) Comprised immunity

7) Blood pressure management

Due to its therapeutic value, the kratom pill has been accepted and used in various counties across the globe. In Europe and America, the drug is used to manage and control pain in patients. In most of the countries, it is a legal medicinal product that is availed to patients in natural health stores, pharmacies and other health facilities. The other advantage of the pill is that it exhibits minimal side effects. Also, there are minimal cases of adverse reactions that have been reported. When taken in the right doses the pill is safe. The drug in pill form has made it easy to determine the dosage and to swallow the pill devoid of bitterness. The drug is readily available and can be purchased online and shipped to your destination.

The interest and attention that this pill made out kratom extracts have attracted over the years confirms its efficiency in the management of human health. Rational use of the drug makes it viable not just being a wonder drug but a very specific medicinal agent that have high therapeutic value. Attractively, the kratom pill remains in the natural state for a long period hence it has a prolonged shelf life.

CHAPTER FIVE: HOW TO PREPARE KRATOM FOR CONSUMPTION

Kratom leaves are normally chewed fresh in the native region after removing the central vein. The dried leaves are also chewed, but it is most preferred when crushed or powdered for easy swallowing. Mixing powdered kratom with water before drinking is quick and easy as well as mixing it with other liquids like milk, kefir or fruit juice. For masking the taste, chocolate milk works better. Powdered kratom can be transformed into a paste for easy swallowing with water, or it can also be mixed with yogurt or applesauce. It can be turned into a capsule. The dried leaves are made into a tea which can be strained and taken. A resin-like extract is prepared by evaporating the water content of kratom tea and can be kept for future use. Little pallets of this extract can be consumed as tea when dissolved in hot water or can be swallowed. Kratom tea can be mixed with other teas like black tea or herbal tea before consumption. Honey or sugar can be added to make it sweeter.

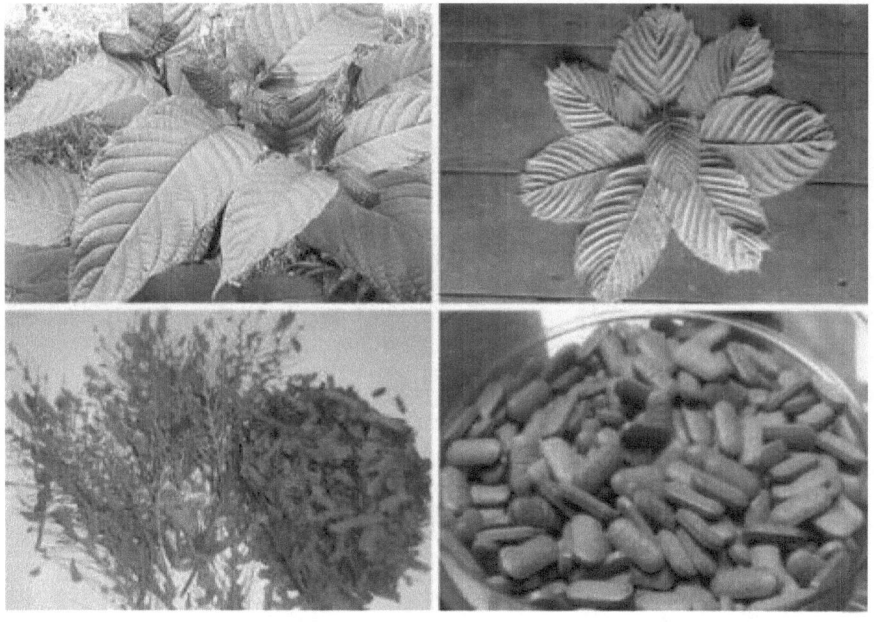

Kratom Leaves in different forms.

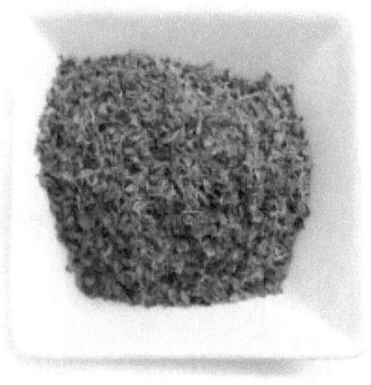

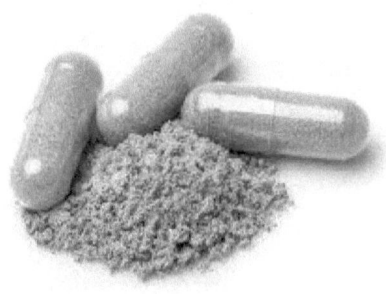

Coarsely Crushed Kratom Leaves

Powdered Kratom Leaves

How to prepare chocolate kratom milkshake

Kratom leaves usually are chewed fresh in the native region after removing the central vein. The dried leaves are also chewed, but it is most preferred when crushed or powdered for easy swallowing. Mixing powdered kratom with water before drinking is quick and easy as well as incorporating it with other liquids like milk, kefir or fruit juice. For masking the taste, chocolate milk works better. Powdered kratom can be transformed into a paste for easy swallowing with water, or it can also be mixed with yogurt or applesauce. It can be turned into capsules. The dried leaves can be transformed into a tea which can be strained and taken. A resin-like extract is prepared by evaporating the water content of kratom tea and can be kept for future use. Little pallets of this extract can be consumed as tea when dissolved in hot water or can be swallowed.

Kratom tea can be mixed with other teas like black tea or herbal tea before consumption. Honey or sugar can be added to make it sweeter.

How to prepare chocolate kratom milkshake

This is the best way of consuming kratom. The chocolate milk covers up the bitterness of kratom and also its viscosity prevents the settling of the kratom to the bottom. Most times, kratom does float on water and also form lumps even after storing it. To avoid this, these steps are to be followed:

Put a dose of powdered kratom into a cup

Add the same volume of chocolate milk like 1-2 tablespoons.

Stir until a homogeneous paste is formed between the liquid and the kratom.

Still, add a few more tablespoons of chocolate milk as you keep storing to form smooth and free of lumps.

Add any remaining milk and stir.

The chocolate kratom is ready for drinking at this point.

How to prepare a powdered kratom paste

Put a dose of kratom powder in an empty cup

Add an equal volume of water as the kratom to make a soft paste. Keep stirring the mixture until the kratom absorbs the water entirely thereby forming a homogeneous paste.

Keep a glass of water separately in a different cup and set aside. As you take an easy to swallow a spoon of the paste, gulp some water to wash the mixture down. Continue to take it like this till the whole paste is finally consumed.

How to prepare kratom powder slurry

Put a powdered kratom into about 7 grams of any beverages or a glass of water

Stir thoroughly until a suspension of the kratom powder is formed. Then gulp as fast as possible to avoid settling of the kratom.

Still, add extra water or beverages to regain any kratom that is stuck to the sides of the cup.

Stir again and drink

Sip a little more juice to remove the bitter taste.

How to make kratom tea

Place about 56 grams of coarsely crushed or ground dried kratom leaves in a pot and add about one liter of water to it.

Boil for 15 minutes

Using a strainer, pour the tea into a bowl. Squeeze the leaves to have most liquids out.

Place the leaves back into the pot and add another liter of water and start boiling again. Repeat the 3rd step after which the leaves are discarded.

Then pour the mixture of the liquids back into the pot and continue boiling to reduce the volume to about 250ml.

How to prepare dried kratom leaves

Dried kratom leaves whether coarsely ground, crushed or whole can be made into powder by using a coffee grinder or kitchen blender to process them at high speed for a few minutes. Though many sellers supply the finely powdered kratom.

CHAPTER SIX- THE HEALTH BENEFITS OF KRATOM

The Health Benefits Of Kratom Powder

Kratom powder is one of the herbs derived from kratom plants. These plants are found in Southeast Asia, and it is being marketed to the U.S. and other countries. This herb has a bitter taste because it contains alkaloid compounds. Thailand people have long used kratom leaves as traditional medicine. The leaves are consumed in any of the following ways: by chewing, made into a tea and processed into powder. Kratom has some benefits for health. The following are some health benefits of Kratom.

Overcoming drug addiction

Rehabilitation clinics most times use kratom to overcome addiction on drugs like opium and morphine addiction. Detoxification is performed in the early stages of rehabilitation to remove the residual toxins of opium or morphine. At this stage will cause some unpleasant symptoms. There is usually a strong desire in patients to return to the consumption of opium or morphine. Therefore, Kratom powder is used to replace those drugs. Kratom is not addictive so that the using can be stopped after the residual toxins of opium out of the patient's body. Due to its effectiveness for Opioid withdrawal, in Thailand, one of the significant uses of kratom is for treating opiate addiction which is a withdrawal problem both for legal use and illegal use of opiate drugs. Unfortunately, consistent use of opiate drug gets the users addicted which is not the desire of the users. Report from many people said that kratom is very efficient for settling this addiction. This is because it possesses alkaloids which act as opiate receptor agonist and so can substitute the opiate drugs, both for opiate withdrawal and for pain medication. After switching to kratom for a given period, people reported that they gradually quit the consumption without having the opiate withdrawal difficulty. That is to say that even though kratom contains opiate receptor agonist, but its pharmacology differs from that of opiate drugs.

Addressing diarrhea

Diarrhea is among the diseases caused by harmful bacteria living in the digestive system. The alkaloids contents in kratom powder are capable of killing the harmful bacteria that live in the digestive system. By destroying the bacteria that causes diarrhea, your disease will be cured.

Increase endurance

Kratom is known rich in antioxidants, especially alkaloids. This substance is believed powerful to increase endurance.

Lowers blood pressure

Kratom contains many alkaloids, one of them is epicatechin. According to some studies, anti oxidant can reduce high blood pressure. It also has been proven by the society of Thailand who uses kratom powder for hypertension for a long time.

Increase energy

Thailand people have long been used kratom as an energy booster. They use it by chewing the leaf of kratom to increase stamina. Stimulant and calming effect caused by kratom make people who consume it feel more fresh and energized.

Overcome muscle pain

Muscle pain is often a result of nerve disorders. Kratom contains several alkaloids that are soothing. The soothing effect is potent to overcome the pain in the muscles. As analgesia, Kratom is very useful in pain treatment. Apart from opium, it is the most effective herb for analgesia available. Lots of people use kratom to relieve pains associated with conditions like fibromyalgia and arthritis.

Overcome depression

Kratom has some alkaloids that are soothing. One of them is mitragynine. This substance is powerful to overcome depression, anxiety, and other psychiatric illnesses.

Sexual stimulant

Thailand people have long been used kratom as medicine to increase sexual arousal. The content of alkaloids in kratom has a stimulant effects and also calming the nerves. This will allow you to control your mind. With a controlled mind, will allow you to have intercourse longer.

Controlling blood sugar levels

Diabetes is often linked with an increase in blood pressure. High sugar levels also lead to a rise in blood viscosity thereby making the pumping blood heavier for the heart. The effect is a rise in blood pressure. The alkaloids content in kratom especially epicatechin is believed to be able to control blood sugar levels and also lower blood pressure. For those of you who have diabetes are very good to consume kratom powder as tea or in the form of capsule.

Recreational purpose

A mixture of kratom leaves, coca cola, ice, and cough syrup knew as 4×100 (a tea-based cocktail) were used among the youths in Southeast Asia during 2011 for recreational purposes.

CHAPTER SEVEN: KRATOM EFFECTS AND DOSAGE

It's hard to pinpoint what are good effects as this is purely subjective. One person may be comfortable with one particular kratom effects, while another person prefers another kind. You can change the type based on your mood. Little Indonesian on mornings when can create a mild relaxing effect and for a heavier hit (like an evening or weekend), a Thai powder like Maeng Da. Kratom effects can do well, though effects are dependent on the person taking it and the type of kratom consumed. The kratom effects when an extract or a blend is taken differs from that when a regular kratom leaf is used.

The minor side effects are vomiting, constipation, nausea. The severe side effects are decreased breathing(respiratory depression), addiction, seizure, and psychosis. Some other side effects are high blood pressure, heart rate, liver toxicity, difficulty with sleep, withdrawal syndrome, death (when taken alone or with other substance).

Kratom, when taken in low-moderate dose, can be stimulating while the high dose can cause sedation because of the stimulant and sedative nature of the active alkaloids. Therefore, the effect varies between individuals or depends on the dosage.

At the stimulant level, the physical strength (maybe or not sexual strength) is accelerated, the mind is much more alert, there will be high motivation to do work especially hard jobs, increase in the mood (that's the antidepressant effect), improved social life. Kratom stimulant effect is a more cognitive effect than a physical impact.

At the Sedative-euphoric level, there is low sensitivity to emotional and physical pains, the overall feeling of comfort, cool look and feel, and pleasant dreamy reverie. There might be sweating and itching, constriction of the pupil, nausea which can subside with relaxation, mixed-state of waking to dream.

Maeng Da Pimps Grade Kratom Effects

This seems to be the new strongest kratom available in the market, though with a trade-off. It has stronger and more intense effects which don't last as long. Maeng Da kratom effects start 20 minutes after consumption but last only 2-3 hours. It is energetic rather than heavy and sedating.

For mild effects: 2 grams

For medium effects: 4-5 grams

For strong effects: 8 - 10 grams

Very strong would be 10 grams +

Maeng Da Kratom effects - if this sounds like something you're interested in, we have a buy kratom section that links to vendors like Arena Ethnobotanicals.

Indonesian Kratom effect

Indonesian kratom (or Indo) gives lighter, more relaxing effects compared to Thai strains. It also has a lighter color & it is cheaper to buy. So, do you need to relax? If you are undergoing a large amount of stress daily, a particular strain of Indonesia kratom may give the desired effects.

The new strains of Indonesian kratom are also available in the market, for example, "super Indo" and "UEI" (Ultra Enhanced Indo). These are Indonesian kratom powder with the combination of either powdered kratom resin or kratom 15x. "Super Indo" to offers the best effects which give better value than the UEI.

Dosage:

5 grams of Indo powder (or crushed leaf): for Mild Effects

8-10 grams of Indo powder (or crushed leaf): Medium Effects

12-15 grams of Indonesian powder: Strong Effects

These are simply a rough guideline. Start with small amounts and work your way up to find your optimum Indo effects.

15x Kratom Effects

This is an extract of kratom in which active alkaloids are isolated for maximum effect with very little material. This product has the possibility of turning into a crumbly mess. I recommend a vendor in the USA that stocks Kratom 15x.

Does:

1-2 grams (although 1 gram may have no effects at all): Mild Effects

3-4 grams: Medium Effects

5-6 grams: Strong Effects

Note that this product is not in any way 15 times stronger more than the regular powder. Instead, it simply means that 15 grams of powder are taken to make 1 gram of extract which explains the ratio.

Thailand Kratom Effects

Thailand kratom is seen as the original as well as the best kratom in the market with much stronger defects than the other strains and last longer. It is a little more expensive when compared with other strains. For strong sedative effects for a connoisseur, this is the one for you.

Effects Associated With Doses (Dosage Guideline)

Depending on the kratom's potency, below are the dosage guideline for different varieties of kratom gotten from Sage Wisdom Botanicals.

Premium Quality Kratom

(oral dosage)

Threshold	2-4 grams
Mild	3-5 grams
Moderate	4-10 grams
Strong	8-15 grams
Very Strong	12-25 grams

Ultra-Potent Kratom

(oral dosage)

Threshold	1-3 grams
Mild	2-4 grams
Moderate	3-7 grams
Strong	6-10 grams
Very Strong	8-16 grams

Kratom Extract

(oral dosage)

Threshold	1 gram
Mild	1-2 grams
Moderate	2-4 grams
Strong	3-6 grams
Very Strong	5-8 grams

Threshold = apparent, but subtle effects

Mild = stimulant-like effects

Moderate = stimulant-like or sedative-euphoric-analgesic effect

Strong = The effects are sedative-euphoric-analgesic and can be too strong for highly sensitive people.

Very Strong = The effects can be sedative-euphoric-analgesic and can be very strong for most individuals.

CHAPTER EIGHT: KRATOM AS A PARTIAL OPIOID AGONIST

What does that mean? Well, for a plant to be an opiate that means it needs to be derived from the opium poppy plant. Opiates are things like heroin, hydrocodone, oxycodone, morphine. Opioids or opioid agonists are any types of drug whether natural or synthetic that bind to the same opioid receptors in the brain, spinal cord, digestive tract, and other areas of the body. For instance, tramadol that's an opioid, Buprenorphine, the main ingredient in Subutex and suboxone that's also an opioid, methadone is an opioid but Kratom is a partial opioid agonist. So it's just a more mild version, and it binds to those opioid receptors similar to but not identical to opiates. It's the herbal supplement that is not as strong as opiates, but it has soothing effects on the receptors. The two main alkaloids that bind to the receptors are

Mitragynine and 7-hydroxymitragynine which is more potent Mitragynine gives it some of the opioid agonist effects as well as some of the stimulating effects and 7-hydroxymitragynine is just a more potent opioid agonist. Since Kratom is an opioid agonist, it can help with opiate withdrawal, pain relief, mood enhancement, muscle tension. It also has anti-inflammatory alkaloids.

Science of opioid withdrawal

When you first start using an opiate or opioid drug it might feel potent. After you use the drug daily for probably a few weeks to a month, you're going to develop what's known as a tolerance that means you need the more of the drug to achieve the same desired effect. After tolerance comes dependence. Physiological dependence is when your neurons now require a certain amount of opioid medication to be healthy. For instance, a painkilling CNS depressant, once you have a dependency, that means that your opioid blood concentrations need to stay at a certain level each day otherwise you're going to experience withdrawal symptoms with symptoms like anxiety, diarrhea, depression, hot and cold flashes, insomnia, stomach discomfort, exhaustion, and even restless leg syndrome. Kratom is, therefore, an herbal remedy that binds to the opioid receptors that when you use enough can stop all withdrawal symptoms and can create a good feeling.

CHAPTER NINE: HOW TO USE KRATOM FOR OPIOID RECOVERY

step one is your transition from your current opiate or opioid to Kratom: You would stop taking the drugs you're addicted to, but that should be after taking it at the usual time and go to sleep at night, then the next morning when you wake up that is when you would start using Kratom so you would use it on an empty stomach. One teaspoon is the starting point. An hour after that's if you still feel like you need more you can take two teaspoons. Always make sure to take it on an empty stomach. Two teaspoons are the moderate dose, but if you're taking capsules, it depends on how big the pill is but try to take about three grams to six grams. Eight, nine or ten grams is excellent but anything above ten grams which is a little over three teaspoons is not advisable but even if you should take it, you would take it around three or four times a day. Find the dosage that helps you the most. Remember, you're not trying to get high off the Kratom you're just trying to feel stabilized, you're trying to feel a relief of withdrawal symptoms and a relief of fatigue and cravings.

Step two is stabilizing the Kratom for one to six weeks depending on your situation:

If you're coming off hydrocodone, oxycodone or heroin or another short acting opioid drugs, then you know you could be stabilized for a week or two if you want and then you could start the taper. If you're on buprenorphine or methadone, any long-acting opioids, it's more beneficial to stabilize on Kratom for about three to four weeks. This is because it takes a long time for the buprenorphine and the methadone to get out of your system especially if you've been on it for several months or years. If you've been on it for years, you might want to stabilize on Kratom for about four or five weeks or something like that because it takes so long for those drugs to come out of your receptors and for your body to get rid of it and detox from it. This will get your body like dependent on the Kratom which is a herbal, less potent, partial opioid agonist.

After step two, the stabilization period then you began a kratom taper. When you taper off opiates or opioids or Kratom or any drug, you could taper off benzodiazepines, or you could taper off caffeine. Whenever you taper off something, you significantly reduce the shock to your body by getting your body used to those lower and lower dosages. So maybe every seven to ten days you reduce your dosage and then gives your body a couple of days to get used to the dose drop and you start to feel normal again. After a few more days you drop back. Along with this creative taper transition method, there's also specific supplements you can take, a particular profile of nutrition, and specific exercise.

CAUTION

Sensitivity to kratom can vary in different individuals and also the can vary with kratom from various sources. Therefore, it is necessary, to begin with, a low dose and gradually increase the dosage until a desirable dose or effect is attained. Do Not consume a strong or a very strong dose the first time a new batch of kratom is being sampled. Individuals that are highly sensitive are advised to take kratom on an empty stomach (that is to wait 3 hours after eating) to avoid nausea when consuming a strong dose. Hypersensitive people are likely to experience adverse reaction like prolonged vomiting when a strong dose is used.